NATURAL REMEDY FOR CANCER

Unlocking Nature's Healing Power: A Comprehensive Guide to Natural Remedies for Cancer

ADOOH MARCEL

Natural Remedy for Cancer

DEDICATION

This book is dedicated to God almighty and my entire family for their unwavering support, boundless encouragement, and profound love they have showered upon me throughout my life and in the course of writing this book. They are the beating heart of my existence, and I want the world to know just how profoundly I appreciate their presence in my journey. And I pray that the almighty God bless them all.

Natural Remedy for Cancer

Copyright 2023 – Adooh Marcel

Natural Remedy for Cancer

Table of Contents

Natural Remedy for Cancer

Natural Remedy for Cancer

Natural Remedy for Cancer

Natural Remedy for Cancer

INTRODUCTION

Natural remedies for cancer refer to alternative treatments and therapies that are derived from natural sources or lifestyle changes and are used alongside or instead of conventional medical treatments. It's important to note that while some natural remedies may have potential benefits, they should never be used as a sole treatment for cancer. Conventional medical treatments, such as surgery, chemotherapy, radiation therapy, and targeted therapies, are the standard of care for most types of cancer.

That said, many people explore natural remedies as complementary approaches to support their overall well-being during cancer treatment. Here are some common natural remedies and approaches often considered in cancer care:

1. **Diet and Nutrition:**
   - A balanced and nutritious diet can help support the immune system and overall health. Some cancer patients turn to specific diets, like the Mediterranean diet, which emphasizes fruits, vegetables, whole grains, and lean proteins.
   - Certain foods like turmeric, green tea, cruciferous vegetables, and medicinal mushrooms (e.g., reishi and maitake) are believed to have anti-cancer properties.
2. **Herbal and Botanical Remedies:**
   - Some herbs and plants, like aloe vera, echinacea, and mistletoe, are used in various forms (capsules, extracts, teas) as complementary treatments.
   - Essiac and Flor Essence are herbal blends often promoted as cancer remedies, but their effectiveness is still a subject of debate.
3. **Mind-Body Practices:**

Natural Remedy for Cancer

- Techniques like meditation, yoga, acupuncture, and massage therapy may help alleviate cancer-related symptoms, reduce stress, and improve quality of life.

4. **Exercise:**
   - Regular physical activity can improve mood, reduce fatigue, and enhance physical well-being during cancer treatment.

5. **Supplements:**
   - Some patients take supplements like vitamin D, omega-3 fatty acids, or coenzyme Q10 to address nutritional deficiencies or support their overall health.

6. **Traditional Chinese Medicine and Ayurveda:**
   - These ancient systems of medicine offer herbal remedies and therapies that some people find beneficial in managing cancer symptoms.

7. **Alternative Therapies:**
   - These include treatments like ozone therapy, hyperthermia, and high-dose vitamin C therapy, which are sometimes used as adjunct therapies in cancer care.

It's crucial to approach natural remedies for cancer with caution and in consultation with a qualified healthcare provider. Natural remedies can have side effects, interactions with conventional treatments, and may not be scientifically proven to treat cancer. Patients should always inform their oncologist about any complementary therapies they are considering to ensure there are no conflicts with their cancer treatment plan.

Ultimately, the best approach for managing cancer is a combination of conventional medical treatments and supportive care, which may include some of the natural remedies mentioned above. Each patient's situation is unique, and treatment decisions should be based on their specific diagnosis and the guidance of their healthcare team.

Natural Remedy for Cancer

CHAPTER ONE
THE ROLE OF NATURAL REMEDIES

Natural remedies can play a supportive role in healthcare and wellness, including in the context of cancer treatment, by addressing various aspects of health and well-being. However, it's important to emphasize that natural remedies should never replace conventional medical treatments for serious conditions like cancer. Their role is typically complementary and supportive. Here are some key roles that natural remedies can play:

1. **Symptom Management**: Natural remedies can help alleviate some of the symptoms and side effects associated with cancer and its treatment. For example, ginger may be used to reduce nausea and vomiting caused by chemotherapy, and acupuncture or massage can help with pain and stress relief.

2. **Improving Overall Health**: A balanced diet, rich in fruits and vegetables, can support overall health and the immune system. Specific foods and supplements may provide essential nutrients that promote general well-being.

3. **Enhancing Quality of Life**: Mind-body practices like meditation and yoga can enhance mental and emotional well-being. They may reduce stress, anxiety, and depression, thereby improving the quality of life for cancer patients.

4. **Strengthening the Immune System**: Some natural remedies, such as certain herbs and supplements, are believed to have immune-boosting properties, potentially helping the body's natural defenses in the fight against cancer.

5. **Managing Side Effects**: Certain natural remedies, like aloe vera or calendula creams, can be used topically to soothe skin irritations and radiation burns caused by cancer treatments.

6. **Complementary Therapies**: Some alternative therapies like acupuncture, chiropractic care, and naturopathy are used alongside

Natural Remedy for Cancer

conventional treatments to support a patient's overall well-being. These therapies should be administered by qualified practitioners.

7. **Psychological and Emotional Support**: Natural remedies, along with counseling and support groups, can help patients and their families cope with the emotional and psychological challenges that often accompany a cancer diagnosis.

8. **Preventative Measures**: Maintaining a healthy lifestyle, including a balanced diet, regular exercise, and stress management, can contribute to cancer prevention by reducing risk factors.

9. **Enhancing Wellness during Survivorship**: Natural remedies and lifestyle changes can be used to promote wellness after cancer treatment is completed. They can help individuals regain strength, reduce the risk of cancer recurrence, and improve their overall health.

It's crucial to approach natural remedies with caution and consult with a healthcare professional, especially when dealing with a serious illness like cancer. Natural remedies can have side effects, interactions with medications, and their effectiveness may vary from person to person. In many cases, the best approach to cancer care is a combination of conventional medical treatments and complementary therapies, all under the guidance of a healthcare team to ensure the safety and well-being of the patient.

DIET AND NUTRITION

Diet and nutrition play a fundamental role in our overall health, and they are particularly important when it comes to cancer prevention, management, and recovery. Here are some key aspects of diet and nutrition in relation to cancer:

1. **Cancer Prevention**:
    - A balanced diet that is rich in fruits, vegetables, whole grains, and lean proteins can reduce the risk of developing certain types of cancer.

Natural Remedy for Cancer

- Consuming a variety of colorful fruits and vegetables provides essential vitamins, minerals, antioxidants, and dietary fiber that support the body's defenses against cancer.

2. **Maintaining a Healthy Weight**:
   - Excess body weight, especially obesity, is a significant risk factor for many cancers, including breast, colon, and kidney cancer. A healthy diet can help individuals maintain an appropriate weight.
3. **Limiting Processed Foods and Sugars**:
   - High consumption of processed foods, sugary beverages, and foods with added sugars has been associated with an increased risk of some cancers. Reducing the intake of these items can contribute to a healthier diet.
4. **Healthy Fats**:
   - Consuming healthy fats, such as those found in nuts, seeds, avocados, and fatty fish, can support overall health. These fats provide essential fatty acids and are linked to a lower risk of certain cancers.
5. **Limiting Red and Processed Meats**:
   - High consumption of red and processed meats has been linked to an increased risk of colorectal cancer. Reducing the intake of these meats and opting for lean protein sources, like poultry and fish, can be beneficial.
6. **Moderate Alcohol Consumption**:
   - Excessive alcohol consumption is associated with an increased risk of certain cancers, including breast, liver, and esophageal cancer. It's advisable to limit alcohol intake or avoid it altogether.
7. **Adequate Hydration**:
   - Staying well-hydrated is important for overall health. Adequate hydration can help flush toxins from the body and support various bodily functions.
8. **Anti-Inflammatory Foods**:

Natural Remedy for Cancer

- Foods with anti-inflammatory properties, such as turmeric, ginger, and berries, may help reduce chronic inflammation, which is associated with the development and progression of some cancers.

9. **Supplements**:
    - Some individuals with cancer may have specific dietary deficiencies, and their healthcare providers may recommend supplements, such as vitamin D or certain minerals, to address these deficiencies.
10. **Customized Diet Plans**:
    - Some cancer patients may benefit from personalized diet plans developed by registered dietitians or nutritionists, taking into account their specific nutritional needs, side effects of treatment, and individual preferences.
11. **Eating During Treatment**:
    - Cancer treatments can often lead to side effects that affect appetite and digestion. In such cases, healthcare providers may recommend modifications to the diet to help manage these issues.

It's essential for cancer patients and individuals looking to reduce their cancer risk to work with healthcare professionals, such as oncology dietitians, to develop a nutrition plan that suits their specific needs. The dietary recommendations may vary based on the type of cancer, treatment phase, and individual circumstances. A well-balanced and nutritious diet can contribute to overall health and support the body's ability to prevent and manage cancer.

THE IMPACT OF DIET ON CANCER

Diet has a significant impact on cancer in several ways, from influencing the risk of developing cancer to affecting the progression and management of the disease. Here are some key aspects of how diet can influence cancer:

Natural Remedy for Cancer

1. **Cancer Risk Reduction**:
   - A healthy and balanced diet can reduce the risk of developing certain types of cancer. This is achieved through the consumption of foods that contain nutrients, antioxidants, and phytochemicals that protect cells from damage and support the immune system.
   - Diets rich in fruits and vegetables, especially those with vibrant colors, provide essential vitamins, minerals, and antioxidants that help to neutralize harmful free radicals and prevent DNA damage.
   - High-fiber foods, like whole grains and legumes, can reduce the risk of colorectal cancer and help maintain a healthy weight.
2. **Weight Management**:
   - Excess body weight and obesity are established risk factors for various cancers, including breast, colon, kidney, and endometrial cancer. A diet that helps maintain a healthy weight can reduce the risk of these cancers.
   - High-calorie, low-nutrient diets can contribute to weight gain and obesity. Consuming nutrient-dense foods and practicing portion control are important for weight management.
3. **Inflammatory Response**:
   - Chronic inflammation is associated with the development and progression of cancer. Diets high in processed foods, added sugars, and unhealthy fats can promote inflammation.
   - Conversely, a diet rich in anti-inflammatory foods, such as turmeric, ginger, and fatty fish, can help mitigate inflammation and potentially reduce cancer risk.
4. **Hormone Regulation**:
   - Some cancers, like breast and prostate cancer, are hormone-sensitive. Diet can impact hormone levels, and certain dietary patterns may promote or inhibit the production and activity of hormones that influence cancer development.

Natural Remedy for Cancer

- For example, diets high in saturated fats and low in fiber can increase estrogen levels, potentially raising the risk of hormone-sensitive cancers.

5. **Reducing Carcinogen Exposure**:
   - The consumption of certain foods, particularly processed and charred meats, has been linked to an increased risk of cancer due to the formation of carcinogens during cooking.
   - Limiting the intake of red and processed meats can reduce exposure to these potential carcinogens.

6. **Alcohol Consumption**:
   - Excessive alcohol consumption is associated with an increased risk of various cancers, including breast, liver, and esophageal cancer. Reducing or eliminating alcohol intake can decrease this risk.

7. **Supporting the Immune System**:
   - Nutrient-rich foods and a well-balanced diet can support a strong immune system, which plays a crucial role in identifying and eliminating abnormal cells that can develop into cancer.

8. **Side Effects and Treatment Tolerance**:
   - During cancer treatment, diet can help manage side effects and improve treatment tolerance. For instance, a soft or bland diet may be recommended for patients with mouth sores, while high-protein diets can support muscle mass during treatment.

It's important to note that while diet can play a significant role in cancer risk reduction and management, it should be part of a comprehensive approach to cancer prevention and care. Lifestyle factors such as physical activity, tobacco and alcohol use, and regular medical check-ups also contribute to cancer prevention. Additionally, individual dietary needs and recommendations can vary based on the type of cancer, its stage, and the specific circumstances of the patient. Consulting with a registered dietitian or healthcare provider can help individuals develop personalized

Natural Remedy for Cancer

dietary strategies to reduce their cancer risk or support their cancer treatment journey.

ANTI-CANCER FOODS AND NUTRIENTS

Certain foods and nutrients are believed to have potential anti-cancer properties, and their consumption is often recommended as part of a balanced and healthful diet to reduce cancer risk. While these foods and nutrients are not a guarantee against cancer, they can contribute to overall well-being and may help in cancer prevention. Here are some examples:

1. **Fruits and Vegetables**:
   - **Berries:** Blueberries, strawberries, and other berries are rich in antioxidants, particularly anthocyanins, which have been associated with reducing cancer risk.
   - **Cruciferous Vegetables:** Broccoli, cauliflower, Brussels sprouts, kale, and cabbage contain compounds like sulforaphane and indole-3-carbinol that may have cancer-fighting properties.
   - **Tomatoes:** Tomatoes are a good source of lycopene, an antioxidant that has been studied for its potential role in reducing the risk of certain cancers, especially prostate cancer.
2. **Whole Grains**:
   - Whole grains like oats, quinoa, and brown rice are high in dietary fiber, which can help reduce the risk of colorectal cancer and support a healthy digestive system.
3. **Fatty Fish**:
   - Fatty fish, such as salmon, mackerel, and sardines, are rich in omega-3 fatty acids. These healthy fats may help reduce inflammation and lower the risk of cancer.
4. **Legumes**:
   - Beans, lentils, and chickpeas are excellent sources of plant-based protein, fiber, and various phytochemicals that can contribute to cancer prevention.

Natural Remedy for Cancer

5. **Nuts and Seeds**:
   - Almonds, walnuts, flaxseeds, and chia seeds provide healthy fats, fiber, and antioxidants that may help reduce cancer risk.
6. **Turmeric**:
   - Curcumin, the active compound in turmeric, has anti-inflammatory and antioxidant properties and is currently being studied for its potential role in cancer prevention and treatment.
7. **Green Tea**:
   - Green tea contains polyphenols, particularly epigallocatechin-3-gallate (EGCG), which are believed to have protective effects against various types of cancer.
8. **Garlic and Onions**:
   - These members of the allium family contain sulfur compounds that may have cancer-fighting properties, particularly in relation to gastrointestinal cancers.
9. **Vitamin D**:
   - Adequate vitamin D levels are associated with a lower risk of certain cancers. You can get vitamin D from sunlight exposure, fortified foods, and supplements.
10. **Antioxidant-Rich Foods**:
    - Foods rich in antioxidants, such as dark chocolate, artichokes, and a variety of colorful fruits and vegetables, can help protect cells from damage by free radicals.
11. **Mushrooms**:
    - Certain mushrooms, like shiitake and reishi, contain compounds that have been studied for their potential anti-cancer effects.
12. **Berberine**:
    - Found in plants like goldenseal and barberry, berberine is a compound under investigation for its potential anti-cancer properties.
13. **Probiotics**:
    - Maintaining a healthy gut microbiome through the consumption of probiotic-rich foods, like yogurt and

Natural Remedy for Cancer

fermented foods, may have a role in supporting the immune system and reducing inflammation, which can influence cancer risk.

It's important to remember that a diet rich in anti-cancer foods and nutrients is just one aspect of a comprehensive cancer prevention strategy. Lifestyle factors, such as regular physical activity, not smoking, and alcohol moderation, also play crucial roles in reducing cancer risk. Additionally, individual dietary recommendations may vary based on factors like age, gender, genetics, and personal health history. If you have concerns about cancer risk or are interested in dietary strategies, consider consulting with a healthcare provider or registered dietitian for personalized guidance.

DIETARY GUIDELINES

Dietary guidelines are evidence-based recommendations provided by health authorities to promote optimal nutrition and well-being for the general population. These guidelines are designed to help individuals make informed and healthy food choices that can contribute to the prevention of chronic diseases, including cancer. While dietary guidelines can vary by country or region, many share common principles. Here are some general dietary guidelines that can support cancer prevention and overall health:

1. **Eat a Variety of Foods**:
   - Consume a wide range of foods from all food groups to ensure a balanced intake of nutrients.
2. **Fruits and Vegetables**:
   - Include a variety of colorful fruits and vegetables in your daily diet. These provide essential vitamins, minerals, and antioxidants that can help reduce the risk of cancer and other diseases.
3. **Whole Grains**:

Natural Remedy for Cancer

- Choose whole grains like whole wheat, oats, brown rice, and quinoa over refined grains. Whole grains are rich in fiber and other nutrients that support overall health.

4. **Protein Sources**:
   - Incorporate a variety of protein sources into your diet, including lean meats, poultry, fish, beans, lentils, tofu, and nuts.

5. **Limit Processed Foods**:
   - Reduce your intake of highly processed foods, which are often high in added sugars, unhealthy fats, and sodium. These foods are associated with an increased risk of cancer and other health issues.

6. **Limit Sugary Drinks**:
   - Minimize consumption of sugary beverages like soda, fruit juices, and energy drinks, as they are linked to an increased risk of obesity and related cancers.

7. **Limit Red and Processed Meats**:
   - Limit the consumption of red meat, such as beef, pork, and lamb, and processed meats like hot dogs and bacon, as they have been associated with an increased risk of colorectal cancer.

8. **Healthy Fats**:
   - Choose healthy fats, such as those found in avocados, nuts, seeds, and olive oil, and limit saturated and trans fats found in fried and processed foods.

9. **Portion Control**:
   - Be mindful of portion sizes to help maintain a healthy weight.

10. **Adequate Hydration**:
    - Drink plenty of water throughout the day to stay well-hydrated.

11. **Limit Alcohol**:

Natural Remedy for Cancer

- If you choose to drink alcohol, do so in moderation. Excessive alcohol consumption is associated with an increased risk of certain cancers.

12. **Salt Reduction**:
    - Reduce salt intake and choose low-sodium options, as high salt consumption is linked to an increased risk of stomach and other cancers.
13. **Food Safety**:
    - Practice safe food handling to prevent foodborne illnesses, which can weaken the immune system and potentially increase cancer risk.
14. **Special Dietary Considerations**:
    - For individuals with specific dietary needs or medical conditions, consult a registered dietitian or healthcare provider for personalized guidance.
15. **Physical Activity**:
    - Combine a healthy diet with regular physical activity to maintain a healthy weight and reduce cancer risk.

It's important to remember that dietary guidelines are intended for the general population and may need to be adjusted for individual circumstances and health conditions. If you have specific concerns about your diet and its impact on cancer prevention or management, consider consulting with a healthcare provider or registered dietitian who can provide personalized recommendations based on your unique needs and goals.

CHAPTER TWO
HERBAL REMEDIES

Herbal remedies, also known as herbal medicine or phytotherapy, involve the use of plant-based substances like leaves, roots, seeds, and extracts to promote health, prevent and manage various ailments, or alleviate symptoms. While some herbal remedies have been used for centuries and have shown promise in certain applications, it's essential to approach them with caution and consult a healthcare professional before using them, especially in the context of serious conditions like cancer. Here are some herbal remedies that have been considered in complementary and alternative medicine:

1. **Echinacea**:
   - Echinacea is often used to boost the immune system and may be taken in the form of capsules, teas, or tinctures. It's believed to help prevent and treat respiratory infections, although its effectiveness is a subject of debate.
2. **St. John's Wort**:
   - St. John's Wort is used for mood disorders, particularly mild to moderate depression. It is available in capsules, teas, and extracts.
3. **Turmeric**:
   - Curcumin, the active compound in turmeric, is known for its anti-inflammatory and antioxidant properties. It is being researched for its potential in cancer prevention and management.
4. **Milk Thistle**:
   - Milk thistle is used to support liver health and may be taken to help protect the liver from damage. It's available in capsule or liquid extract form.

Natural Remedy for Cancer

5. **Aloe Vera**:
   - Aloe Vera gel is used topically to soothe skin irritations, including burns. Some people also consume aloe vera juice, though its safety and effectiveness are still debated.
6. **Garlic**:
   - Garlic is believed to have cardiovascular benefits and some anti-cancer properties. It can be consumed raw, as a supplement, or in cooked dishes.
7. **Ginger**:
   - Ginger is often used to alleviate nausea, particularly in cancer patients undergoing chemotherapy. It can be consumed as ginger tea or supplements.
8. **Mistletoe**:
   - Mistletoe extract is used in some parts of the world as an alternative cancer therapy, often in conjunction with conventional treatment. Its effectiveness is controversial, and it should only be used under medical supervision.
9. **Ginseng**:
   - Ginseng is thought to enhance energy and reduce fatigue. It is available in various forms, including capsules, powders, and teas.
10. **Saw Palmetto**:
    - Saw palmetto is used in herbal medicine to manage symptoms of benign prostatic hyperplasia (enlarged prostate). It is typically taken as a dietary supplement.
11. **Green Tea**:
    - Green tea is rich in antioxidants and is believed to have potential health benefits, including cancer prevention. It can be consumed as a beverage or in supplement form.
12. **Arnica**:
    - Arnica is used topically to reduce inflammation and ease muscle pain and bruises. It is available in creams, gels, and ointments.

Natural Remedy for Cancer

It's important to exercise caution and informed decision-making when using herbal remedies. Not all herbal products are regulated or tested for safety and efficacy, and interactions with medications are possible. Before using herbal remedies, it is advisable to consult with a healthcare provider, especially if you have a pre-existing medical condition or are undergoing conventional cancer treatment. Additionally, it's essential to inform your healthcare team about any herbal remedies you plan to use, as they can impact your overall treatment plan.

OVERVIEW OF HERBAL MEDICINE

Herbal medicine, also known as phytotherapy or botanical medicine, is a traditional and holistic approach to healing and wellness that involves the use of plant-based remedies to prevent, treat, or manage various health conditions. Herbal medicine has been practiced for centuries in different cultures around the world and continues to be a significant part of complementary and alternative medicine today. Here's an overview of herbal medicine:

1. **Historical Roots**: Herbal medicine has a long history, dating back to ancient civilizations such as the Chinese, Ayurvedic, Native American, and traditional African systems. These systems have developed intricate knowledge of plants and their healing properties over generations.
2. **Plant-Based Remedies**: Herbal medicine relies on the use of various plant parts, including leaves, roots, stems, flowers, and seeds. These plant materials can be used in their natural form or processed into different preparations, such as teas, tinctures, capsules, extracts, and topical applications.
3. **Holistic Approach**: Herbal medicine is often grounded in a holistic view of health, considering the interconnectedness of the body, mind, and spirit. Practitioners of herbal medicine typically address the root causes of health issues and aim to restore balance and vitality.

Natural Remedy for Cancer

4. **Traditional Knowledge**: Traditional herbalists or healers possess extensive knowledge of local plants and their therapeutic uses. This knowledge is often passed down through oral traditions and apprenticeships.
5. **Modern Herbalism**: In contemporary times, herbal medicine has evolved and integrated with modern scientific research. This combination of traditional wisdom and scientific understanding is sometimes referred to as "phytopharmacology."
6. **Potential Benefits**: Herbal medicine is used for a wide range of health concerns, including the management of common ailments like colds, insomnia, and digestive issues. Some herbs are also explored for their potential in preventing and managing chronic conditions like diabetes and cancer.
7. **Safety and Efficacy**: While many herbal remedies have demonstrated therapeutic effects, the safety and efficacy of herbal medicines can vary. Some herbs can interact with medications or have side effects, and the quality of herbal products may not always be assured. It's crucial to consult with a qualified herbalist or healthcare provider when using herbal remedies, especially for serious conditions.
8. **Regulation**: The regulation of herbal medicines varies by country. In some regions, herbal products are regulated as dietary supplements, while in others, they are classified as traditional medicines. Regulatory agencies may establish safety and quality standards for these products.
9. **Research and Evidence**: The field of herbal medicine is actively evolving, with ongoing research into the therapeutic properties of specific plants and their active compounds. Clinical studies are conducted to assess the safety and efficacy of herbal remedies.
10. **Integration with Conventional Medicine**: Some healthcare providers integrate herbal medicine into their practice, often in conjunction with conventional medical treatments. This integrative approach is known as complementary or integrative medicine.

It's important to approach herbal medicine with care and seek

Natural Remedy for Cancer

guidance from trained practitioners or healthcare professionals, especially when dealing with serious or chronic health conditions. The use of herbal remedies should be well-informed, considering individual health needs and potential interactions with medications. As with any form of healthcare, open communication with your healthcare team is essential to ensure safe and effective treatment.

HERBAL TEAS AND SUPPLEMENTS

Herbal teas and supplements are popular forms of herbal remedies that people use for a wide range of purposes, from relaxation and stress relief to supporting overall health. Some herbal teas and supplements are believed to have potential health benefits, including the prevention and management of various conditions. Here's an overview of herbal teas and supplements:

HERBAL TEAS:

1. **Chamomile Tea**:
   - Chamomile tea is known for its soothing and calming properties. It is often used to alleviate stress, anxiety, and sleep disturbances. Some people also use it for digestive issues.
2. **Peppermint Tea**:
   - Peppermint tea can help relieve digestive discomfort, including indigestion and irritable bowel syndrome (IBS). It has a refreshing flavor and may help reduce nausea.
3. **Ginger Tea**:
   - Ginger tea is used to alleviate nausea and motion sickness. It also has anti-inflammatory properties and is sometimes used for pain relief.
4. **Lemon Balm Tea**:
   - Lemon balm tea is believed to have calming and mood-improving effects. It is often used to reduce stress and anxiety.

Natural Remedy for Cancer

5. **Echinacea Tea**:
   - Echinacea tea is consumed to boost the immune system and may help prevent or alleviate colds and upper respiratory infections.
6. **Hibiscus Tea**:
   - Hibiscus tea is rich in antioxidants and is believed to support heart health and help lower blood pressure.
7. **Nettle Tea**:
   - Nettle tea is used to alleviate allergy symptoms and hay fever. It's also consumed for its potential diuretic effects.
8. **Dandelion Tea**:
   - Dandelion tea may have diuretic properties and is used to support liver health. It can also be consumed for its potential digestive benefits.

HERBAL SUPPLEMENTS:

1. **Ginkgo Biloba**:
   - Ginkgo biloba supplements are believed to improve cognitive function and memory. They may be used by some individuals for age-related cognitive decline.
2. **Saw Palmetto**:
   - Saw palmetto supplements are commonly used by men to manage symptoms of benign prostatic hyperplasia (enlarged prostate).
3. **Garlic Supplements**:
   - Garlic supplements may help support heart health and reduce cholesterol levels. Garlic is also believed to have anti-inflammatory and antimicrobial properties.
4. **Milk Thistle**:
   - Milk thistle supplements are used to support liver health and are believed to protect the liver from damage caused by toxins and medications.

Natural Remedy for Cancer

5. **Valerian Root**:
   - Valerian root supplements are used to promote relaxation and improve sleep quality. They are often used as a natural remedy for insomnia and anxiety.
6. **Black Cohosh**:
   - Black cohosh supplements are used by some women to alleviate menopausal symptoms like hot flashes and mood swings.
7. **St. John's Wort**:
   - St. John's Wort supplements are believed to have antidepressant properties and are used by some people to manage mild to moderate depression.
8. **Turmeric/Curcumin**:
   - Turmeric supplements, often containing the active compound curcumin, are used for their anti-inflammatory and antioxidant properties. They are explored for various health benefits, including reducing inflammation and managing chronic diseases.

It's important to exercise caution when using herbal teas and supplements, as they can interact with medications and have potential side effects. Consult with a healthcare provider or a registered herbalist before using herbal products, especially if you have pre-existing medical conditions or are taking medications. Additionally, be sure to obtain herbal products from reputable sources to ensure their quality and purity.

CHAPTER THREE
SUPPLEMENTS

Dietary supplements are products that contain one or more dietary ingredients (such as vitamins, minerals, herbs, amino acids, enzymes, or other substances) that are intended to supplement one's diet. These supplements come in various forms, including pills, capsules, powders, liquids, and gummies. They are typically used to fill nutrient gaps, support overall health, and address specific nutritional needs. Here is an overview of dietary supplements:

1. **Multivitamins and Multiminerals**:
   - Multivitamin and multimineral supplements provide a combination of essential vitamins and minerals that may be missing from one's diet. They are often used as a general nutritional insurance policy.
2. **Vitamin Supplements**:
   - These supplements are used to address specific nutrient deficiencies. Common examples include vitamin D, vitamin C, vitamin B-complex, and vitamin E supplements.
3. **Mineral Supplements**:
   - Minerals like calcium, magnesium, iron, and zinc are available in supplement form. They are often used to meet increased requirements, such as during pregnancy or for specific health conditions.
4. **Omega-3 Fatty Acids**:
   - Omega-3 supplements, typically sourced from fish oil or algae, are taken for heart health, reducing inflammation, and supporting brain function.
5. **Probiotics**:
   - Probiotic supplements contain live beneficial bacteria and yeasts that support gut health and the balance of the gut microbiome.

Natural Remedy for Cancer

6. **Herbal and Botanical Supplements**:
   - These supplements contain plant-based ingredients, such as herbs, roots, and extracts. They are used for various purposes, including immune support, stress relief, and managing specific health conditions.
7. **Amino Acids**:
   - Amino acid supplements, such as branched-chain amino acids (BCAAs), are used by athletes and bodybuilders to support muscle growth and recovery.
8. **Antioxidants**:
   - Antioxidant supplements, like coenzyme Q10 (CoQ10) and alpha-lipoic acid, are believed to help protect cells from damage caused by free radicals.
9. **Collagen Supplements**:
   - Collagen supplements are used for skin health, joint support, and to promote hair and nail growth.
10. **Weight Management Supplements**:
    - These supplements, such as green tea extract and conjugated linoleic acid (CLA), are marketed for weight loss and fat metabolism.
11. **Joint Health Supplements**:
    - Supplements like glucosamine and chondroitin sulfate are used to support joint health and alleviate arthritis-related symptoms.
12. **Plant-Based Supplements**:
    - Plant-based supplements, including those made from spirulina, chlorella, and wheatgrass, are consumed for their nutrient-rich properties.
13. **Fiber Supplements**:
    - Fiber supplements, such as psyllium husk, are taken to support digestive health and alleviate constipation.
14. **Energy and Performance Supplements**:
    - Supplements like caffeine, creatine, and electrolyte products are used to enhance athletic performance and energy levels.

Natural Remedy for Cancer

15. **Specialized Nutritional Supplements**:
    - These supplements are designed for specific groups, such as prenatal vitamins for pregnant women, iron supplements for individuals with anemia, and calcium and vitamin D for postmenopausal women.

It's important to note that dietary supplements are not meant to replace a balanced diet or serve as a substitute for proper nutrition. In many cases, the best way to obtain essential nutrients is through a well-balanced diet. Additionally, dietary supplements should be used cautiously and under the guidance of a healthcare provider. They can have potential side effects, interactions with medications, and may not be necessary for individuals with a balanced and varied diet. Always consult with a healthcare professional before starting any new dietary supplement regimen, especially if you have specific health concerns or medical conditions.

MIND-BODY TECHNIQUES

Mind-body techniques are practices that focus on the connection between mental and emotional processes and physical health. These techniques emphasize the importance of a holistic approach to well-being and have been used to promote relaxation, reduce stress, and support overall health. They are often considered complementary or integrative therapies when used in conjunction with conventional medical treatments. Here are some mind-body techniques:

1. **Meditation**:
    - Meditation involves focusing one's attention and eliminating the stream of thoughts that may be crowding the mind. It can help reduce stress, improve concentration, and promote emotional well-being. Various meditation techniques, such as mindfulness meditation and transcendental meditation, are practiced.

Natural Remedy for Cancer

2. **Yoga**:
   - Yoga is a mind-body practice that combines physical postures, breathing exercises, and meditation. It is known for improving flexibility, strength, balance, and relaxation. Different forms of yoga, such as Hatha, Vinyasa, and Bikram, are available.

3. **Tai Chi**:
   - Tai Chi is a Chinese martial art that involves slow, flowing movements and deep breathing. It is often used to improve balance, flexibility, and relaxation. Tai Chi is suitable for people of all ages and fitness levels.

4. **Pilates**:
   - Pilates is a physical fitness system that focuses on core strength, flexibility, and overall body conditioning. It can help improve posture, reduce back pain, and enhance physical and mental well-being.

5. **Breathing Exercises**:
   - Deep breathing techniques, such as diaphragmatic breathing and the 4-7-8 technique, can promote relaxation and reduce stress. These exercises are often used in yoga, meditation, and mindfulness practices.

6. **Progressive Muscle Relaxation**:
   - This technique involves systematically tensing and then relaxing different muscle groups, promoting physical and mental relaxation. It can help reduce muscle tension and stress.

7. **Biofeedback**:
   - Biofeedback uses electronic monitoring to provide individuals with real-time information about physiological functions like heart rate, blood pressure, and muscle tension. It can help individuals learn to control these functions and reduce stress responses.

8. **Guided Imagery**:

Natural Remedy for Cancer

- Guided imagery involves the use of mental imagery to create a sense of relaxation and well-being. It is often used to manage pain, reduce anxiety, and improve mood.

9. **Hypnotherapy**:
   - Hypnotherapy is the use of guided relaxation and focused attention to achieve a heightened state of awareness and suggestibility. It is sometimes used to address psychological and emotional issues.
10. **Art and Music Therapy**:
    - Art and music therapy involve creative expression to address emotional, psychological, and physical well-being. These therapies can be particularly helpful in managing stress and promoting self-expression.
11. **Mindfulness-Based Stress Reduction (MBSR)**:
    - MBSR is a structured program that combines mindfulness meditation and yoga to reduce stress and improve emotional well-being. It has been used in various healthcare settings.

Mind-body techniques are often considered safe and can be used as part of a broader strategy to support mental and physical health. They may be particularly helpful in managing conditions where stress and emotional well-being play a significant role, such as anxiety, depression, and chronic pain. If you are interested in using mind-body techniques, consider seeking guidance from trained instructors or therapists who can provide appropriate instruction and support for your specific needs.

STRESS REDUCTION

Stress reduction is a crucial aspect of maintaining overall health and well-being, and it can be especially important for individuals dealing with cancer or other serious health issues. Chronic stress can negatively impact the body's ability to heal and cope with illness.

Natural Remedy for Cancer

Here are some strategies for stress reduction, which can be beneficial for cancer patients:

1. **Mind-Body Techniques**:
   - As mentioned earlier, mind-body techniques such as meditation, yoga, tai chi, deep breathing exercises, and mindfulness can help reduce stress and promote relaxation. These practices are often integrated into cancer care programs to improve emotional well-being.
2. **Counseling and Support**:
   - Professional counseling or participation in support groups can provide a safe space to express feelings, fears, and concerns. Talking with a therapist or connecting with others who are going through similar experiences can help alleviate emotional stress.
3. **Physical Activity**:
   - Engaging in regular physical activity, as permitted by the individual's health condition, can reduce stress and improve mood. Even light exercise, such as walking, can be beneficial.
4. **Expressive Arts**:
   - Art, music, and other forms of creative expression can serve as outlets for emotions and stress relief. Art therapy and music therapy can be particularly helpful in this context.
5. **Relaxation Techniques**:
   - Techniques like progressive muscle relaxation, guided imagery, and visualization can help individuals relax and manage stress.
6. **Stress Management Programs**:
   - Some cancer centers offer stress management programs that include a combination of relaxation techniques, cognitive-behavioral therapy, and coping strategies to help patients manage the stress associated with cancer.
7. **Time Management**:

Natural Remedy for Cancer

- Effective time management can reduce stress by helping individuals prioritize important tasks and allocate time for rest and relaxation.

8. **Healthy Lifestyle Choices**:
   - Maintaining a balanced diet, getting enough sleep, and avoiding excessive caffeine and alcohol can support stress reduction. A healthy lifestyle is a foundation for coping with stress.

9. **Social Support**:
   - Family and friends can provide emotional support and practical assistance, reducing the burden of cancer-related stress. Open and honest communication with loved ones can help strengthen these bonds.

10. **Limiting Exposure to Stressors**:
    - Identify and limit exposure to sources of stress whenever possible. This may include setting boundaries, minimizing stressful situations, and seeking support from others.

11. **Professional Help**:
    - If stress becomes overwhelming or leads to persistent anxiety or depression, it may be beneficial to seek the guidance of a mental health professional or counselor who specializes in stress management and coping with chronic illness.

12. **Spiritual or Mindfulness Practices**:
    - For some individuals, engaging in spiritual practices or mindfulness-based activities can provide a sense of inner peace and comfort, reducing stress and promoting a positive outlook.

Stress reduction techniques should be tailored to the individual's preferences and needs. What works best may vary from person to person. Cancer patients should work closely with their healthcare team to develop a stress management plan that aligns with their medical treatment and personal circumstances. Reducing stress can have a positive impact on overall health and can enhance the

Natural Remedy for Cancer

individual's ability to cope with the challenges of cancer and its treatment.

MEDITATION AND MINDFULNESS

Meditation and mindfulness are powerful mind-body techniques that can be used to reduce stress, promote emotional well-being, and improve overall health. They are particularly valuable for cancer patients, as they can help individuals cope with the emotional and physical challenges of the disease. Here's an overview of meditation and mindfulness:

MEDITATION:

Meditation is a practice that involves focused attention and a quieting of the mind. There are various meditation techniques, but they all share the goal of promoting relaxation and inner peace. For cancer patients, meditation can provide the following benefits:

1. **Stress Reduction**: Meditation helps reduce stress and anxiety, which are common emotional responses to a cancer diagnosis and treatment.
2. **Emotional Well-Being**: Regular meditation practice can improve emotional well-being, boost mood, and reduce symptoms of depression.
3. **Pain Management**: Some cancer patients use meditation to manage pain and discomfort, as it can alter the perception of pain and enhance the body's natural pain-relief mechanisms.
4. **Sleep Improvement**: Meditation can promote better sleep, helping cancer patients manage sleep disturbances often associated with the disease and its treatment.
5. **Enhanced Coping Skills**: Meditation helps individuals develop coping skills and resilience in the face of the challenges presented by cancer.

MINDFULNESS:

Natural Remedy for Cancer

Mindfulness is a specific form of meditation that involves being fully present in the moment, accepting one's thoughts and feelings without judgment, and developing an awareness of the present experience. For cancer patients, mindfulness offers several advantages:

1. **Stress Reduction**: Mindfulness-based stress reduction (MBSR) programs are often used in cancer care to help patients reduce stress and improve emotional well-being.
2. **Pain Management**: Mindfulness-based techniques can help individuals cope with pain and discomfort more effectively.
3. **Emotional Resilience**: Mindfulness practices can enhance emotional resilience and coping abilities, allowing cancer patients to navigate the emotional challenges of their diagnosis and treatment.
4. **Enhanced Quality of Life**: Mindfulness can improve overall quality of life by promoting acceptance, emotional balance, and a sense of well-being.
5. **Reduction in Anxiety and Depression**: Mindfulness-based therapies have been shown to reduce symptoms of anxiety and depression in cancer patients.

Both meditation and mindfulness can be practiced through various methods, including:

- **Guided Meditation**: Meditation sessions led by an instructor, either in person or through audio recordings.
- **Breath Awareness Meditation**: Focusing on the breath to quiet the mind and promote relaxation.
- **Body Scan Meditation**: A technique that involves paying attention to physical sensations and areas of tension in the body.
- **Loving-Kindness Meditation**: Cultivating feelings of compassion and kindness towards oneself and others.
- **Mindfulness-Based Stress Reduction (MBSR)**: A structured program that combines mindfulness meditation with stress reduction techniques.

Natural Remedy for Cancer

Cancer patients interested in meditation and mindfulness should consider the following:

- Seek guidance from trained instructors or therapists who have experience working with individuals dealing with cancer.
- Participate in structured programs or classes specifically designed for cancer patients, which are often available at cancer treatment centers.
- Practice regularly to experience the full benefits of these techniques.

Integrating meditation and mindfulness into a cancer care plan can be a valuable component of holistic well-being. They offer tools for managing the emotional and physical challenges that come with a cancer diagnosis and its treatment.

YOGA AND TAI CHI

Yoga and Tai Chi are mind-body practices that encompass physical postures, breathing techniques, and meditation. They can provide numerous benefits for cancer patients, including improved physical and emotional well-being. Here's an overview of both practices:

YOGA:

Yoga is a holistic discipline that combines physical postures (asanas), controlled breathing (pranayama), and meditation to promote physical and mental health. For cancer patients, yoga offers several advantages:

1. **Physical Wellness**: Yoga can improve flexibility, strength, and balance, which are crucial for cancer patients, especially if they are dealing with physical limitations or post-operative recovery.
2. **Stress Reduction**: Yoga helps reduce stress, anxiety, and promotes relaxation, making it a valuable tool for emotional well-being during cancer treatment.

Natural Remedy for Cancer

3. **Pain Management**: Some yoga poses and techniques can help individuals manage cancer-related pain, discomfort, and muscle tension.
4. **Improved Sleep**: Yoga practices can promote better sleep, helping cancer patients manage insomnia and sleep disturbances.
5. **Enhanced Coping Skills**: Through meditation and mindfulness aspects, yoga can help individuals develop resilience and coping skills to deal with the emotional challenges of cancer.
6. **Quality of Life**: Regular yoga practice can lead to an improved overall quality of life, as it supports emotional balance and a sense of well-being.

Cancer patients should consider the following when practicing yoga:

- Consult with healthcare providers before starting a new yoga practice, especially if there are any physical limitations or restrictions.
- Seek out specialized yoga classes or instructors experienced in working with cancer patients. Some cancer centers offer tailored yoga programs.
- Choose a yoga style that is appropriate for the individual's fitness level and health condition. Gentle or restorative yoga may be more suitable for some patients.

TAI CHI:

Tai Chi, often referred to as "meditation in motion," is a Chinese martial art that involves slow, flowing movements and deep, rhythmic breathing. It is known for its meditative and therapeutic qualities. For cancer patients, Tai Chi offers numerous benefits:

1. **Physical Balance and Coordination**: Tai Chi enhances balance, flexibility, and coordination, which are valuable for individuals managing physical challenges related to cancer.

Natural Remedy for Cancer

2. **Stress Reduction**: The slow, deliberate movements and focused breathing in Tai Chi help reduce stress and promote emotional well-being.
3. **Pain Management**: Tai Chi can help individuals cope with chronic pain and muscle tension often associated with cancer and its treatment.
4. **Improved Sleep**: Regular Tai Chi practice may improve sleep quality, reducing sleep disturbances common in cancer patients.
5. **Enhanced Emotional Resilience**: Tai Chi can enhance emotional resilience and provide a sense of well-being, helping patients navigate the emotional aspects of their diagnosis and treatment.

Cancer patients should consider the following when practicing Tai Chi:

- Consult with healthcare providers before starting Tai Chi, especially if they have physical limitations or specific health concerns.
- Join Tai Chi classes led by qualified instructors, especially those experienced in working with individuals dealing with cancer.
- Start with gentle Tai Chi forms and progress at a pace that suits individual physical abilities and health conditions.

Both yoga and Tai Chi can be valuable additions to a comprehensive cancer care plan, promoting physical and emotional well-being. They offer tools to manage the emotional and physical challenges associated with cancer and its treatment. Individuals should work with healthcare providers to determine the best practice for their specific needs and medical conditions.

Natural Remedy for Cancer

CHAPTER FOUR
PHYSICAL ACTIVITY

Physical activity is an important component of cancer care and can play a significant role in improving the physical and emotional well-being of cancer patients. Engaging in regular exercise can have numerous benefits, even during and after cancer treatment. Here's an overview of physical activity for cancer patients:

BENEFITS OF PHYSICAL ACTIVITY FOR CANCER PATIENTS:

1. **Improved Physical Fitness**: Regular exercise can enhance strength, flexibility, and endurance, which are essential for managing the physical challenges of cancer and its treatment.
2. **Stress Reduction**: Physical activity can reduce stress, anxiety, and depression. Exercise promotes the release of endorphins, which are natural mood elevators.
3. **Pain Management**: Some forms of exercise, such as gentle stretching and strength training, can help manage cancer-related pain and discomfort.
4. **Enhanced Immune Function**: Regular physical activity may boost the immune system, supporting the body's natural defenses against illness.
5. **Weight Management**: Maintaining a healthy weight can reduce the risk of complications and improve overall health. Exercise is an important component of weight management.
6. **Reduced Fatigue**: Physical activity can help reduce cancer-related fatigue and increase energy levels.
7. **Improved Sleep**: Regular exercise can improve sleep quality and reduce sleep disturbances, which are common among cancer patients.
8. **Enhanced Coping Skills**: Engaging in physical activity can improve emotional resilience and coping abilities, helping patients navigate the emotional challenges of cancer.

Natural Remedy for Cancer

9. **Bone Health**: Weight-bearing exercise can help maintain bone density, which is important for cancer patients who may be at risk of bone-related complications.

TYPES OF EXERCISE FOR CANCER PATIENTS:

The type and intensity of exercise should be tailored to an individual's specific health condition, treatment status, and fitness level. Here are some forms of exercise that may be suitable for cancer patients:

1. **Aerobic Exercise**: Activities like walking, cycling, and swimming can improve cardiovascular fitness and overall endurance.
2. **Strength Training**: Resistance exercises using light weights or resistance bands can enhance muscle strength and reduce muscle atrophy.
3. **Flexibility and Stretching**: Stretching exercises can improve flexibility, reduce muscle tension, and enhance joint mobility.
4. **Yoga**: Yoga combines physical postures, controlled breathing, and meditation, providing a holistic approach to physical and emotional well-being.
5. **Tai Chi**: Tai Chi's slow, flowing movements and deep breathing promote balance, flexibility, and relaxation.
6. **Pilates**: Pilates exercises can improve core strength, flexibility, and posture.

CONSIDERATIONS FOR PHYSICAL ACTIVITY:

Cancer patients should consider the following when engaging in physical activity:

- Consult with healthcare providers before starting a new exercise regimen, especially if there are any specific health concerns or physical limitations.
- Seek guidance from exercise professionals or trainers experienced in working with cancer patients.

Natural Remedy for Cancer

- Start with gentle exercise forms and gradually increase intensity as tolerated.
- Listen to the body and rest when needed. Fatigue is common during cancer treatment, and it's important to prioritize rest and recovery.

**Benefits of physical activity extend beyond cancer treatment. It can improve overall health and quality of life for cancer survivors. Patients should work closely with their healthcare team to determine the most appropriate and safe exercise plan based on their individual needs and medical conditions.

EXERCISE AND ITS ROLE IN CANCER PREVENTION

Exercise plays a significant role in cancer prevention by reducing the risk of developing various types of cancer. Engaging in regular physical activity and maintaining a healthy lifestyle can have a positive impact on your overall health and well-being. Here's how exercise contributes to cancer prevention:

1. Weight Management: Maintaining a healthy weight is one of the most critical factors in cancer prevention. Obesity is associated with an increased risk of several types of cancer, including breast, colon, kidney, and endometrial cancer. Regular exercise helps control body weight by burning calories and maintaining a healthy balance between energy intake and expenditure.

2. Reduced Inflammation: Chronic inflammation is a risk factor for cancer development. Regular physical activity can help reduce chronic inflammation in the body, which may contribute to a decreased risk of certain cancers.

3. Improved Digestive Health: Physical activity can help maintain a healthy digestive system, reducing the risk of colorectal cancer. Regular exercise can promote regular bowel movements and prevent conditions like constipation, which may increase the risk of colorectal cancer.

Natural Remedy for Cancer

4. Hormone Regulation: Some cancers, such as breast and prostate cancer, are influenced by hormones. Exercise can help regulate hormone levels and reduce the risk of hormone-related cancers.

5. Enhanced Immune Function: Regular exercise can enhance the immune system's ability to detect and destroy abnormal cells, including those that could potentially become cancerous.

6. Better Metabolic Health: Exercise can improve insulin sensitivity and regulate blood sugar levels. Conditions like type 2 diabetes are associated with an increased risk of certain cancers, and exercise can help prevent diabetes.

7. Detoxification: Physical activity can promote sweating, which is one way the body eliminates toxins and waste products. Effective detoxification can help protect against cancer development.

8. Reduced Breast Cancer Risk: Studies have suggested that regular physical activity, particularly during adolescence and early adulthood, can reduce the risk of breast cancer.

9. Prevention of Skin Cancer: While excessive sun exposure is a primary risk factor for skin cancer, regular exercise can help maintain a healthy immune system and overall well-being, which may indirectly contribute to cancer prevention.

10. Psychological Benefits: Exercise has significant psychological benefits, reducing stress, anxiety, and depression. These emotional and mental health benefits can indirectly support cancer prevention, as chronic stress and emotional disturbances are linked to an increased cancer risk.

11. Promoting Healthy Behaviors: Engaging in regular exercise often leads to the adoption of other healthy behaviors, such as a

Natural Remedy for Cancer

balanced diet and not smoking, further reducing the risk of cancer.

To reap the full benefits of exercise in cancer prevention, it's recommended to aim for at least 150 minutes of moderate-intensity aerobic activity or 75 minutes of vigorous-intensity aerobic activity per week, along with muscle-strengthening activities on two or more days a week. It's essential to consult with a healthcare provider before starting a new exercise routine, especially if you have underlying health conditions or have been inactive for an extended period. Additionally, it's important to combine regular exercise with a well-balanced diet and other healthy lifestyle choices for the most effective cancer prevention strategy.

RECOMMENDED EXERCISE ROUTINES

Recommended exercise routines for cancer prevention and overall health can vary based on an individual's fitness level, age, and specific health goals. However, the American Cancer Society and other health organizations offer general guidelines for exercise that can help reduce the risk of cancer and improve overall well-being. Here are some recommended exercise routines for cancer prevention:

1. Cardiovascular (Aerobic) Exercise:

- Aim for at least 150 minutes of moderate-intensity aerobic exercise or 75 minutes of vigorous-intensity aerobic exercise per week. You can break this time into smaller sessions throughout the week.
- Examples of moderate-intensity activities include brisk walking, swimming, and cycling at a pace that elevates your heart rate and makes you breathe harder but still allows for conversation.
- Vigorous-intensity activities might include running, fast cycling, or intense aerobics, where you should be breathing hard and only able to say a few words at a time.

Natural Remedy for Cancer

- Incorporate a variety of activities to keep your routine interesting and to engage different muscle groups. This could include dancing, playing sports, or using exercise machines.

2. Strength Training:

- Include muscle-strengthening activities on at least two days a week. These exercises can help improve muscle mass, bone density, and metabolic health.
- Strength training exercises may involve lifting weights, using resistance bands, or performing bodyweight exercises like push-ups, squats, and lunges.
- Focus on all major muscle groups, including the legs, chest, back, shoulders, and core.

3. Flexibility and Stretching:

- Regularly include stretching exercises to maintain flexibility and improve joint mobility. Flexibility exercises are especially important as we age.
- Stretch all major muscle groups to prevent stiffness and enhance your range of motion.

4. Balance and Coordination:

- Incorporate balance and coordination exercises to improve stability and prevent falls, especially as you get older.
- Activities like Tai Chi and yoga can help with balance and coordination while providing stress-reduction benefits.

5. Lifestyle Incorporation:

Natural Remedy for Cancer

- Incorporate physical activity into your daily routine. This can include taking the stairs instead of the elevator, walking or biking for short errands, or standing up and moving around during prolonged periods of sitting.
- Include active breaks at work, such as standing up and stretching every hour.

6. Stay Hydrated and Wear Appropriate Gear:

- Staying hydrated is important during exercise. Drink water before, during, and after physical activity, especially in warm weather.
- Wear comfortable and appropriate workout clothing and footwear to prevent injury and discomfort.

7. Consult a Healthcare Provider:

- If you have any underlying health conditions, are new to exercise, or have specific concerns related to your health and cancer prevention, consult with a healthcare provider or exercise specialist before starting a new exercise routine.

It's important to remember that consistency is key. Start slowly and gradually increase the duration and intensity of your workouts to prevent injury. Listen to your body, and if you experience any unusual symptoms or discomfort during exercise, consult with a healthcare provider.

Ultimately, the best exercise routine is one that you enjoy and can maintain over the long term. This will help ensure that physical activity becomes a regular part of your lifestyle and contributes to cancer prevention and overall well-being.

Natural Remedy for Cancer

CHAPTER FIVE
ALTERNATIVE THERAPIES

Alternative therapies, also known as complementary or integrative therapies, are non-conventional approaches to healthcare that are used alongside or in conjunction with conventional medical treatments. While they are not typically used as primary cancer treatments, some cancer patients may choose to incorporate alternative therapies to manage symptoms, improve their overall well-being, and support their conventional treatment. It's essential to discuss these therapies with your healthcare team and make informed decisions. Here are some alternative therapies that are sometimes used in cancer care:

1. Acupuncture:

- Acupuncture involves the insertion of thin needles into specific points on the body to help alleviate pain, nausea, and other side effects of cancer treatment.

2. Massage Therapy:

- Massage can provide relaxation, reduce stress, and relieve muscle tension. It may also help manage pain and improve overall well-being.

3. Aromatherapy:

- Aromatherapy uses essential oils and scents to promote relaxation, alleviate anxiety, and enhance emotional well-being.

Natural Remedy for Cancer

4. Mind-Body Techniques:

- These include practices like meditation, yoga, tai chi, and guided imagery, which can help manage stress, improve emotional well-being, and promote relaxation.

5. Herbal Remedies:

- Some herbal supplements and botanicals are used to support cancer patients. Examples include mistletoe, astragalus, and ginseng. However, it's crucial to use these under the guidance of a knowledgeable practitioner, as they may interact with conventional treatments or have side effects.

6. Dietary Supplements:

- Certain dietary supplements, such as high-dose vitamins and minerals, are sometimes used to boost the immune system or alleviate treatment side effects. It's essential to consult with a healthcare provider to ensure safety and effectiveness.

7. Homeopathy:

- Homeopathic remedies involve the use of highly diluted substances to stimulate the body's natural healing responses. They are often used to address symptoms like nausea, pain, and fatigue.

8. Energy Healing:

- Energy healing therapies, including Reiki and therapeutic touch, aim to balance the body's energy and promote relaxation. They are sometimes used to complement cancer care.

Natural Remedy for Cancer

9. Traditional Chinese Medicine (TCM):

- TCM includes practices like herbal medicine, acupuncture, and qigong. It is used to manage symptoms, improve energy flow, and support overall well-being.

10. Naturopathic Medicine: - Naturopathic practitioners use a range of natural treatments, including herbal medicine, dietary counseling, and lifestyle recommendations, to support health and well-being.

11. Chiropractic Care: - Chiropractic adjustments may be used to alleviate pain, discomfort, and improve physical well-being during cancer treatment.

12. Therapeutic Music and Art: - Music therapy and art therapy are creative approaches that can provide emotional support, stress reduction, and a sense of well-being for cancer patients.

It's crucial to keep the following points in mind when considering alternative therapies:

- Consult with your healthcare team: Always discuss your intentions to use alternative therapies with your oncologist or healthcare provider. They can help you make informed decisions and ensure that the chosen therapies are safe and do not interfere with your conventional cancer treatment.
- Choose qualified practitioners: If you decide to explore alternative therapies, seek practitioners who are licensed and experienced in their respective fields.
- Be aware of potential interactions: Some alternative therapies, herbal supplements, and dietary supplements may interact with

Natural Remedy for Cancer

conventional treatments or have side effects. Inform your healthcare team about everything you are using.

- Focus on evidence-based approaches: While some alternative therapies have shown promise in managing symptoms and promoting well-being, it's essential to rely on evidence-based practices to ensure their safety and effectiveness.
- Keep an open line of communication: Maintaining open and transparent communication with your healthcare team is crucial for a well-rounded approach to cancer care. They can provide guidance and monitor your progress throughout your treatment.

ACUPUNCTURE

Acupuncture is a traditional Chinese medical practice that involves inserting thin needles into specific points on the body to stimulate energy flow and promote healing. While it is not a primary cancer treatment, acupuncture is sometimes used as a complementary therapy to help manage cancer-related symptoms and improve overall well-being in cancer patients. Here's an overview of acupuncture and its potential benefits in cancer care:

1. Pain Management:

- Acupuncture can help alleviate cancer-related pain, including pain from tumors, surgery, chemotherapy, or radiation therapy. It may also be useful for managing neuropathic pain and musculoskeletal discomfort.

2. Nausea and Vomiting:

- Some cancer patients experience nausea and vomiting as side effects of chemotherapy or radiation therapy. Acupuncture has been shown to reduce the severity and frequency of these symptoms, helping patients tolerate their treatment better.

Natural Remedy for Cancer

3. Fatigue:

- Cancer-related fatigue is a common and often debilitating symptom. Acupuncture can improve energy levels and reduce the profound tiredness that many cancer patients experience.

4. Anxiety and Stress:

- Acupuncture has a relaxing effect and can help reduce anxiety and stress, which are common emotional responses to a cancer diagnosis and treatment.

5. Improved Sleep:

- Many cancer patients struggle with sleep disturbances. Acupuncture may promote better sleep quality and alleviate insomnia.

6. Immune System Support:

- Acupuncture is believed to support the immune system and help the body's natural healing mechanisms.

7. Improved Overall Well-Being:

- Many cancer patients find that acupuncture enhances their overall sense of well-being and helps them cope with the emotional and physical challenges of cancer.

8. Reduced Medication Dependency:

- Acupuncture may help reduce the need for pain medications and antiemetics, leading to a lower risk of medication-related side effects and dependency.

Natural Remedy for Cancer

9. Minimized Treatment Side Effects:

- When used in conjunction with cancer treatments, acupuncture may help mitigate some of the side effects, making the treatment process more manageable.

10. Individualized Treatment: - Acupuncture treatments are highly individualized, with practitioners tailoring the therapy to the specific needs and symptoms of each patient.

It's essential to keep the following points in mind when considering acupuncture as a complementary therapy in cancer care:

- **Consult with Your Healthcare Team**: Always discuss your intention to use acupuncture with your oncologist or healthcare provider. They can provide guidance, ensure safety, and ensure that it does not interfere with your conventional cancer treatment.
- **Choose a Qualified Acupuncturist**: Seek a licensed acupuncturist with experience working with cancer patients. They should be knowledgeable about the specific needs and potential complications that may arise during cancer treatment.
- **Be Informed**: Ask your acupuncturist to explain the treatment plan, potential benefits, and any possible risks or side effects. Understand what to expect from each session.
- **Monitor Progress**: Maintain open communication with your healthcare team and acupuncturist throughout your treatment. This will ensure that the treatment is safe and effective.

Acupuncture, when used in conjunction with conventional cancer care, may offer benefits in managing symptoms and improving overall well-being. However, it is essential to approach it as a complementary therapy and work closely with healthcare

Natural Remedy for Cancer

professionals to develop a comprehensive care plan.

AROMATHERAPY

Aromatherapy is a holistic and complementary therapy that involves the use of essential oils, aromatic compounds derived from plants, to promote physical, emotional, and mental well-being. Aromatherapy is sometimes used as a complementary therapy in cancer care to manage cancer-related symptoms and enhance the overall quality of life for patients. Here's an overview of aromatherapy and its potential benefits in cancer care:

1. Stress Reduction:

- Aromatherapy can help reduce stress, anxiety, and emotional tension, which are common responses to a cancer diagnosis and treatment. Certain essential oils, such as lavender and chamomile, are known for their calming effects.

2. Pain Management:

- Some essential oils, like peppermint and eucalyptus, have analgesic properties that may help alleviate cancer-related pain, discomfort, and muscle tension.

3. Nausea and Vomiting:

- Aromatherapy may help manage chemotherapy-induced nausea and vomiting. Essential oils such as ginger and citrus oils can be used to alleviate these symptoms.

4. Improved Sleep:

- Patients experiencing sleep disturbances or insomnia may benefit from the relaxing and sedative effects of certain essential oils.

Natural Remedy for Cancer

Lavender, cedarwood, and ylang-ylang are examples of essential oils that can promote better sleep.

5. Emotional Well-Being:

- Aromatherapy can enhance emotional well-being by promoting relaxation, reducing anxiety, and providing a sense of comfort and emotional support.

6. Enhanced Quality of Life:

- Many cancer patients report an improved overall quality of life when they incorporate aromatherapy into their care plan. The pleasant scents and therapeutic properties of essential oils can enhance their well-being.

7. Immune Support:

- Some essential oils, like tea tree and eucalyptus, have antimicrobial properties that can support the immune system and reduce the risk of infection.

8. Enhanced Concentration and Focus:

- Aromatherapy can improve mental clarity and concentration, which may be particularly beneficial for cancer patients experiencing "chemo brain" or cognitive difficulties.

9. Individualized Treatment: - Aromatherapy can be personalized to meet the specific needs and symptoms of each patient. Different essential oils and blends may be used for different purposes.

Natural Remedy for Cancer

When considering aromatherapy in cancer care, keep the following in mind:

- **Consult with Your Healthcare Team**: Always discuss your intention to use aromatherapy with your oncologist or healthcare provider. They can provide guidance, ensure safety, and verify that it does not interfere with your conventional cancer treatment.
- **Choose High-Quality Essential Oils**: Use high-quality, pure essential oils from reputable sources to ensure safety and effectiveness.
- **Patch Test**: Perform a patch test on a small area of skin to check for potential allergic reactions or skin sensitivities before applying essential oils topically.
- **Dilution**: Essential oils are highly concentrated and should be properly diluted in carrier oil when applied to the skin to prevent skin irritation or allergic reactions.
- **Inhalation Methods**: Aromatherapy can be administered through inhalation methods, such as diffusers or inhalers, in addition to topical application.
- **Individual Responses**: Keep in mind that individual responses to aromatherapy can vary. What works well for one person may not have the same effect on another.

Aromatherapy, when used thoughtfully and in consultation with healthcare professionals, can offer a natural and non-invasive way to manage cancer-related symptoms, reduce stress, and enhance overall well-being. It should be approached as a complementary therapy in the context of comprehensive cancer care.

Natural Remedy for Cancer

CHAPTER SIX
DETOXIFICATION

Detoxification, often referred to as "detox," is a process by which the body eliminates or neutralizes toxins and harmful substances. While detoxification has gained popularity as a health practice, it's important to understand its limitations and potential risks, especially in the context of cancer care. Here's an overview of detoxification and its relevance to cancer patients:

1. Natural Detoxification Mechanisms:

- The human body has a natural detoxification system that includes the liver, kidneys, digestive system, and skin. These organs work to process and eliminate toxins and waste products from the body.

2. Detox Diets and Practices:

- Detox diets and practices typically involve the consumption of specific foods, supplements, or the use of therapies such as colon cleansing, saunas, or fasting. The aim is to assist the body's natural detoxification processes.

3. Detox and Cancer Care:

- For cancer patients, the use of detox diets or practices is a subject of debate. While some people turn to detoxification as a way to support their overall health during cancer treatment, it's essential to consider several factors:
- **Potential Risks**: Some detox practices may be risky for cancer patients, particularly those undergoing treatment. Fasting or strict detox diets can lead to malnutrition, compromised immune function, and reduced energy levels, which may be harmful during cancer treatment.

Natural Remedy for Cancer

- **Interaction with Treatment**: Certain detox supplements or practices may interfere with cancer treatments, reduce their effectiveness, or exacerbate side effects. It's crucial to consult with your healthcare team before attempting any detox regimen.
- **Lack of Scientific Evidence**: Many detox practices lack scientific evidence to support their effectiveness. Some products or programs may make bold claims without proper validation.
- **Consultation with Healthcare Providers**: If a cancer patient is considering a detox regimen, it's imperative to discuss it with their oncologist or healthcare provider. They can provide guidance and ensure it aligns with the patient's specific treatment and health condition.

4. Support for Natural Detoxification:

- Instead of extreme detox regimens, cancer patients are often advised to support their body's natural detoxification mechanisms through a well-balanced diet, staying hydrated, and engaging in moderate physical activity. These healthy habits can help the body process toxins and eliminate waste products efficiently.

5. Individualized Approaches:

- Each cancer patient's needs and circumstances are unique. Therefore, any potential detoxification efforts should be individualized and monitored by healthcare professionals to ensure safety and effectiveness.

In summary, while detoxification has gained popularity as a means of promoting health, it's important to exercise caution and skepticism, especially for cancer patients. Extreme detox practices or unproven supplements may carry risks and should be approached with the guidance and approval of healthcare providers. The focus for cancer patients should be on supporting the body's natural detoxification mechanisms through a healthy and balanced lifestyle,

Natural Remedy for Cancer

in consultation with their healthcare team.

SAFETY AND PRECAUTIONS

Safety and precautions are critical considerations when exploring natural remedies, alternative therapies, and complementary practices in the context of cancer care. While many of these approaches can offer benefits, it's essential to ensure they are used safely and effectively. Here are some key safety tips and precautions to keep in mind:

1. Consult with Your Healthcare Team:

- Always discuss any natural remedies, complementary therapies, or alternative treatments with your oncologist or healthcare provider. They can provide guidance, assess potential interactions with your conventional treatment, and ensure the chosen approach is safe and appropriate for your specific health condition.

2. Choose Qualified Practitioners:

- Seek licensed and experienced practitioners when considering complementary therapies like acupuncture, massage therapy, or herbal medicine. Verify their qualifications and credentials.

3. Medication and Treatment Interactions:

- Be aware that some natural remedies and supplements may interact with conventional cancer treatments, reducing their effectiveness or causing unwanted side effects. Inform your healthcare team of everything you are using, including supplements.

4. Be Skeptical of Bold Claims:

Natural Remedy for Cancer

- Be cautious of treatments or products that make sweeping claims about curing cancer. While some natural remedies can support cancer care, there is no scientifically proven "magic cure" for cancer.

5. Quality and Safety of Supplements:

- If you're using dietary supplements, ensure they are of high quality, pure, and from reputable sources. Consider supplements only under the guidance of a healthcare provider.

5. Individualized Approaches:

- Recognize that each cancer patient's needs and responses to therapies are unique. What works for one person may not work for another. Focus on an individualized approach to cancer care.

6. Monitor for Side Effects:

- Keep an eye out for any unexpected or adverse side effects when using natural remedies or complementary therapies. Report them to your healthcare provider.

7. Avoid Extreme Measures:

- Extreme detox diets, fasting, or other rigorous practices can be risky for cancer patients, potentially leading to malnutrition or reduced energy levels. Consult with your healthcare team before attempting any extreme measures.

8. Holistic Lifestyle Approaches:

- Consider a holistic approach to cancer care, which includes a balanced diet, regular exercise, stress management, and emotional support. These factors play a significant role in overall well-being.

Natural Remedy for Cancer

9. Follow Recommended Guidelines:

- Adhere to recommended guidelines for specific natural remedies or practices. For instance, if using herbal medicine, follow dosage instructions from qualified practitioners.

11. Transparency and Communication:

- Maintain open communication with your healthcare team. Let them know about any natural remedies, therapies, or dietary changes you're considering or have implemented.

10. Research and Education:

- Educate yourself about the natural remedies and complementary therapies you're interested in. Look for reputable sources of information and consider the scientific evidence behind these approaches.

In summary, safety and precautions are paramount when considering natural remedies and complementary practices in cancer care. Always consult with your healthcare team, use qualified practitioners, and prioritize open communication to ensure that the chosen approaches are safe, effective, and aligned with your overall cancer treatment plan.

CHAPTER SEVEN
CONCLUTION

Natural remedies can be a valuable complement to conventional cancer treatments, helping manage symptoms, improve overall well-being, and support the healing process. When exploring natural remedies for cancer, it's important to approach them with careful consideration and under the guidance of healthcare professionals. Here's a summary of key points regarding natural remedies for cancer:

1. Role of Natural Remedies:

- Natural remedies, also known as complementary or alternative therapies, are used alongside conventional cancer treatments to manage symptoms, alleviate side effects, and enhance overall well-being. They are not typically used as standalone cancer treatments.

2. Diet and Nutrition:

- Diet plays a crucial role in cancer care. A well-balanced and nutritious diet can support the immune system, promote healing, and help manage treatment-related side effects.

3. Herbal Remedies:

- Herbal medicine involves the use of plant-based remedies to manage cancer-related symptoms. It's important to use herbs under the guidance of qualified practitioners to avoid potential interactions and side effects.

Natural Remedy for Cancer

4. Supplements:

- Dietary supplements may be used to support specific health needs during cancer care. Consult with healthcare providers to ensure their safety and effectiveness.

5. Mind-Body Techniques:

- Mind-body techniques such as meditation, yoga, and stress reduction practices can help reduce stress, improve emotional well-being, and enhance the body's healing response.

6. Physical Activity:

- Regular exercise and physical activity play a crucial role in cancer prevention and support overall health during cancer treatment.

7. Alternative Therapies:

- A variety of alternative therapies, including acupuncture, massage therapy, aromatherapy, and more, can help manage cancer-related symptoms and provide emotional support. Consult with healthcare providers to ensure safety.

8. Safety and Precautions:

- When using natural remedies or complementary therapies, it's essential to consult with healthcare providers, choose qualified practitioners, and prioritize safety. Monitor for side effects and maintain open communication with your healthcare team.

Incorporating natural remedies into your cancer care plan can be a valuable addition to conventional treatments, helping to address both physical and emotional aspects of cancer. However, it's crucial to

Natural Remedy for Cancer

approach these remedies with careful consideration, individualization, and under the guidance of healthcare professionals to ensure their safety and effectiveness in your specific situation.

IMPORTANCE OF HOLISTIC HEALTH

Holistic health, often referred to as holistic or integrative medicine, is an approach to healthcare that considers the whole person—mind, body, and spirit—as a dynamic and interconnected system. It recognizes that health and well-being are influenced by various factors, including physical, emotional, social, environmental, and spiritual aspects. Here's an overview of the importance of holistic health:

1. Comprehensive Care:

- Holistic health takes a comprehensive view of an individual's health, considering not only physical symptoms but also emotional, social, and spiritual aspects. This approach allows healthcare providers to address all dimensions of health.

2. Prevention and Wellness:

- Holistic health places a strong emphasis on preventive care and maintaining overall well-being. It encourages healthy lifestyle choices, such as a balanced diet, regular exercise, and stress management, to prevent illness and promote longevity.

3. Individualized Care:

- Holistic health recognizes that each person is unique, with their own health challenges, goals, and preferences. Healthcare providers work with patients to create personalized treatment plans that align with their specific needs.

Natural Remedy for Cancer

4. Emotional and Mental Health:

- Emotional and mental well-being are integral components of holistic health. This approach addresses conditions like stress, anxiety, and depression, providing strategies and therapies to enhance emotional and mental health.

5. Alternative and Complementary Therapies:

- Holistic health embraces a wide range of alternative and complementary therapies, such as acupuncture, massage, meditation, and herbal medicine. These therapies can be used to support conventional medical treatments and manage symptoms.

6. Mind-Body Connection:

- Holistic health acknowledges the strong connection between the mind and body. Emotional and psychological factors can impact physical health, and vice versa. Addressing this mind-body connection is central to holistic care.

7. Supportive Care for Chronic Conditions:

- Holistic health is particularly valuable for individuals with chronic conditions, including cancer. It offers a range of supportive therapies that help manage symptoms and improve quality of life.

8. Patient Empowerment:

- Holistic health encourages patients to actively participate in their healthcare decisions. It empowers individuals to take responsibility for their health and make informed choices.

Natural Remedy for Cancer

9. Complementary to Conventional Medicine:

- Holistic health does not replace conventional medicine but complements it. It integrates evidence-based practices with complementary and alternative therapies to provide well-rounded care.

10. Holistic Lifestyle:

- Holistic health encourages a holistic lifestyle that encompasses not only healthcare choices but also healthy diet, regular physical activity, and a positive, balanced approach to life.

11. Focus on Quality of Life:

- Holistic health places a strong emphasis on enhancing the quality of life, even in the presence of illness. It aims to improve physical, emotional, and mental well-being, providing comfort and support.

In summary, holistic health is an approach to healthcare that recognizes the importance of addressing the whole person, rather than just isolated symptoms or conditions. It promotes individualized, preventive care, emphasizes emotional and mental well-being, and empowers patients to actively participate in their healthcare. Holistic health complements conventional medicine and offers a well-rounded approach to promoting health and well-being.

Natural Remedy for Cancer